NO MAN'S LAND:

A Caregiver's Survival Guide

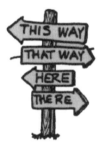

SUSAN G. MILLER, M. S.

*Living with Alzheimer's
and Related Dementias*

*Volume Two
of the Unplanned Journey Trilogy*

NO MAN'S LAND:
A Caregiver's Survival Guide
Copyright © 2003 Susan G. Miller

All rights reserved. No part of this book may be reproduced by any means, except in context of review, without prior written permission from the publisher. For more information, or to order additional copies, contact:

Kaleidoscope Kare Press
110 Pheasant Run Road
Wilton, CT 06897

(203) 762-5713

A portion of the proceeds from the sale of this book
will be donated to the Alzheimer's Association.

Library of Congress Cataloging-in-Publication Data

Miller, Susan G., 1943-
    No man's land : a caregiver's survival guide : living with alzheimer's and related dementias / Susan G. Miller.— 1st ed.
    p. cm.
    ISBN 0-9679584-5-8
    1. Alzheimer's disease—Popular works. 2. Caregivers—Popular works. I. Title.
    RC523.2 .M554 2003
    362.1'96831—dc21   2002151366
                                                                       CIP

Cover design by Chuck Hathaway, Mendocino Graphics

Book production by Cypress House
www.cypresshouse.com

Printed in Canada
1 3 5 7 9 8 6 4 2

To my husband, Don,
whose kindness continues to shine through.

To my daughter, Laura,
who gave us the gift we needed to ease our journey,

our precious granddaughters,
Madeleine Louise and Lauren Elizabeth.

To my son, Brian,
whose sensitivity and support have meant the world to me.

Foreword

- ♠ Imagine coming home from the store and laying your package down, only to find it gone thirty minutes later and nowhere to be found.

- ♠ Imagine looking for your favorite cereal in the morning, not finding it anywhere, and only later, when you go to do a load of wash, do you find it.

- ♠ Imagine living with your spouse of many years, only to wake one day and find he has turned into your child.

- ♠ Imagine thinking you are living in a house of cards, or that you are imagining it all, or that perhaps it's just a dream and you'll soon awaken.

If you are a caregiver to someone suffering from Alzheimer's or related dementias, you'll have no trouble imagining this, because you've lived it. I invite you to follow along on my journey, and I hope my words will validate, support, and comfort you.

If you are not a caregiver my words will seem strange to you, and you might even wonder about my mental condition. I invite you to follow along with the intent of better understanding and appreciating the journey caregivers travel.

Contents

INTRODUCTION xi

Answer 1
No Man's Land 3
Feel 5
Vows 6
Ordinary Couple 7
Not Ordinary 8
Robbed 8
Identity 9
Fades 9
Letting Go... 10
Tips: The Caregiver's Lexicon 12

TRANSITION 15
New Role 18
Slipped 19
Domino Effect 20
He's Gone 21
Shell 22
Lost It 23
Next Time 24
Door 24
Point of No Return 25
Props 25
Tips on Transition 26

IMPACT	28
The New Me	31
Defining Moments	32
Martha Stewart	33
Lost Voice	34
Long Hours	35
Survivor	36
Seasons	36
Vacation	37
Brief Moment	37
Option	38
Sunglasses	38
Frozen Solid	39
Vacation	39
Vacation for One	40
Differentiation	40
Just Happened	41
Fantasy	42
Morphed	43
Slow Down	44
Meltdowns	45
Meltdown Day	46
Context	46
Shattered	47
Fantasy	47
Change of Heart	48
Quality of Life	50
Amazed	51
Tips Tried and True	52

HEALTHCARE PROFESSIONALS ... 55
Disconnect ... 59
Advice ... 60
Message ... 60
Don't Get It ... 61
Face ... 62
Who's The Stupid One Here? ... 63
My Therapist: Best Interest ... 64
My Therapist: Luxury ... 65
Lunar Moon ... 66
Zen ... 67
Guru ... 68
Charts ... 69
Another Expert ... 70
White Coats... ... 71
Imagination ... 72
Changing ... 73
Truth ... 74
Understanding ... 75
Surprised ... 76
Dilemma ... 77
Rehearsal ... 78
Peace ... 79
Experts ... 79
Tips for Communicating with Healthcare Professionals   80

RELATIONSHIPS ... 82
Weekend Away ... 85
Brief Moments ... 85

Sigh	86
Talk Over	87
My Daughter and I	88
My Son and I	89
Watch	90
Special Child	91
My Heart	92
Maddie	93
Lauren	94
Message to Friends	95
Work	96
Support Group	97
Mirror Reflection…	98
Strong…	99
Questions with No Answers	100
Why?	100
Bets	101
Surprise	102
Needs	103
Tips on Relationships	104
CONCLUSION	106
Unguarded Moment	107
Trust	107
Terrain	108
Fine	109
About the Author	110

Introduction

Alzheimer's Tidal Wave Feared

That's what the headlines of a national newspaper read... claiming that within the next twenty-five years thousands of baby boomers will begin to develop the disease, pushing the current number of 4 million to epidemic proportions. For once, the press couldn't get me riled up with dramatic headlines designed to sell papers. While their figures were accurate, we were already ahead of the baby boomers by a number of years. In 1998, after many years of increasingly strange behavior for which no medical expert could find a reason, my husband was, at age fifty-five, diagnosed with Alzheimer's. The headline simply left me feeling numb and sad for those whose future would be forever altered. I hoped they were enjoying today, the time they have before this horrific disease, which steals one's identity day by day, depletes family savings, and exhausts caregivers, became a reality. Researchers are continuing to explore many avenues in hopes of eradicating this dreaded disease, but until then, many more will make the unplanned journey that my husband and I are taking.

If someone had told me BA (Before Alzheimer's, as I often refer to that part of my life these days) that I would write a book, I'd have laughed and said they had me mixed up with someone else—perhaps the famous author, Sue Miller. Writing had become my therapy, a place to express my deepest feelings; something I did just for myself. At a 1999 Alzheimer's Conference in Connecticut where I was speaking, in a moment of sheer audacity, I shared a few poems to illustrate a point. The audience response, both, at the moment and afterwards, was what propelled me to publish my first book, *Uplanned Journey: Understanding the Itinerary*, which chronicled the emotional roller coaster ride I encountered upon diagnosis and embarkation upon a new way of life.

For simplicity's sake I've chosen to look at the illness in three stages: beginning, middle, and end. For a more definitive understanding, refer to the works of Barry Reisberg, M.D. My intention was, and is, to serve as an advocate for sufferers of the illness, and their caregivers. Once my book was published, people began asking me when my next book was coming out. I found myself pushing the release date farther and farther ahead. On one hand, I had much of the material and format completed, but on the other hand, some strange force was holding me back. Eventually, I realized that the strange force was myself. My second book has been difficult, and reflects my own anguish and chaos as I wrestled with my husband's continued decline and the conflicting emotions it evoked in me. It's never pleasant to come face to face with one's limitations and dark side, but for those of us who are caregivers it comes with the territory. Caregiving, by and of itself, is a tremendous task, but when one is caregiving for someone whose essence disappears slowly before one's eyes, the task becomes almost beyond love and endurance. The coping skills that had served me well no longer sufficed. Everything I believed about myself was turned upside down as the demands of the illness stole more of my time and changed the essence of who I was. My reluctance to share this with readers reflected my own reluctance to come to terms with what was happening to us as a couple and as individuals. Finally, through trial and error, I learned to ease up on the demands I made of myself, and not to criticize myself so harshly, which allowed me to move on and finish the book.

Having completed the beginning stage—acceptance and acclimation—it seemed as if suddenly we were propelled into the middle stage, which marked the end of denial and put to rest the belief that we could beat it. Once again I felt somewhat unprepared, like a stranger visiting my own life. *No Man's Land: A Caregiver's Survival Guide*, begins with my husband's transition into middle stage. I have tried to capture honestly the painful feelings I experienced as I navigated the issues of middle stage. In some ways it was like starting all over again, adapting to new behaviors and changing needs that required a new way of living, and to my husband's continual decline. Middle stage demands a lot from caregivers: it's a time of assessment, of planning for the future, and of creating an environment conducive to the needs of both parties. This translated, for me, into a different set of coping skills: a shift in mindset, a need to develop boundaries defining what I could do, what I was willing to do, and what was simply beyond my endurance; and continuing to keep my husband safe, healthy, and stimulated.

Answer

I have been asked by
Well-wishers, friends, strangers,
People afflicted with Alzheimer's,
Even family,
Why we would go public with our story.
Why are we so involved with the Alzheimer's Association?
Why would I write a book sharing my innermost feelings?
Why do I lecture on the subject?
Why did we agree to appear on CBS's "Eye on America?"
I ponder these questions and hope they are asked
Out of simple curiosity
And not with a hidden message or innuendo.
I have no reply except,
Until you are dealing with a disease so feared
People don't want to hear or speak about it,
A disease that until recently Medicare did not reimburse,
Until you fear that there is a possibility
That your children could share a similar fate,
Until you have sat through one too many jokes
About Alzheimer's or senior moments,
Until you have experienced the pain of friends
Distancing themselves,
No answer will make sense.

What I can tell you is:
This is not a disease to be ashamed of,
This is not a disease to be hidden away,
This is not a disease to leave families to suffer in silence,
Or deplete their financial and emotional resources,
This is a disease that needs to be understood, not feared,
And one of the ways to accomplish this
Is to go public with your journey.

No Man's Land

In the beginning our journey was complicated.
We did not know what direction to follow.
Be in a study?
Sign up for controversial gene therapy?
Change medications and go with the newest?
Move and be closer to our children?
There was no itinerary to follow, yet we stumbled through,
Getting off track every now and then
But never getting lost
I would like to say we sailed through,
But that would be a lie.
It was difficult
Shock, like never known before,
Sleepless nights,
Monumental disbelief,
Anger and all that comes with it,
And just as we were getting used to it,
Thought we had it mastered,
We entered no man's land... middle stage,
Feeling like, perhaps, we had taken a wrong turn
Missed a sign, taken a detour.
But we had not; we were right on time, right on course,
And all the old emotions returned,
But just not with such force. How different it is,

A whole new road map
Calling for a different navigational system.
Now I look back and think beginning stage was a snap,
But my support group members' stories and reactions
remind me of the truth.
Middle stage feels like a holding pattern
between the beginning and the end,
Not as good as the past,
but not as bad as the future—
No man's land.

Feel

I feel like a garden plant with a bushel placed over it.
I feel as if I am on a one-way road that is endless.
I feel a sense of injustice for my husband
Stricken too soon for a cure.
I feel sorrow for our children losing their father far too early,
Sadness for our grandchildren
Who will know him only through our memories.
I feel the collective pain and exhaustion
Of all families dealing with this illness.
I feel comforted by those who have gone before me,
Illuminating the way.
I feel the kindness of strangers, the judgment of others.
I feel the hope of the research scientists
Who strive to eradicate this disease.
I feel thankful for the strength of the human spirit.
I feel grateful for those who have supported us
Along the way.
I feel the gratitude of those that have read my words
And let me know it helped them.
I feel the promise of tomorrow,
Even if it is not what I hoped it to be.

Vows

For richer or poorer, for better or worse
In sickness and health, till death do us part.
Vows taken long ago
When we were young and full of dreams,
When they were just words, part of a ceremony,
When the future loomed bright,
When Alzheimer's was referred to as senile dementia
And just for the elderly,
When surely nothing bad would befall us,
When love was the answer to all of life's problems.
Now thirty-eight years later and a diagnosis of Alzheimer's,
The past holds more days than the future,
And we have become part of a grim statistic
Four million strong,
Our life together fast forwarded and condensed,
Both at the same time, giving it a surreal quality,
And the belief that nothing bad would befall us
Shattered like our dreams, along with the knowledge
That love is not the answer, only a part.
For richer or poorer, for better or worse
In sickness and health, till death do us part
This is our journey.

Ordinary Couple

We were an ordinary couple once,
Like you,
Your neighbors,
Your friends,
Or perhaps even your parents.
An ordinary couple,
Nothing wrong with that,
Married for many years,
Raised a couple of children
Buried a parent,
Lost a friend,
Had our share of disappointments and triumphs,
Moments of anger when we entertained
The possibility of leaving
But stayed instead to continue to weave the tapestry
Of what we were together,
An ordinary couple.

Not Ordinary

We sit across from each other at the restaurant,
Laughing, sharing an intimacy.
We lie on the beach enjoying the sun, clearly on vacation.
We shop for baby clothes, delighting in our purchases,
Obviously thrilled to be grandparents.
We look ordinary
Like any other middle-aged couple enjoying themselves,
But we are not ordinary.
We have been fast-forwarded into a time and place
That was to be years away.

Robbed

We have been robbed as surely as if a thief
Made his way into our home
And confiscated our most prized possessions
We have been robbed of a relationship,
A life, a future, and our dreams
We have been robbed
But there is no one to report the crime to,
No insurance form to fill out,
No retribution or condolences to be given.

Identity

He has lost his identity of corporate businessman,
Financial expert, husband,
Replaced by a childlike innocence
And an old man's demeanor.
I have lost my identity of career woman,
Fun-loving friend, wife,
Replaced by caregiver, cook, and mother.

Fades

Caregiving, in the beginning, is seductive,
Shielding one from knowing what they have taken on,
And if the illness is short in duration,
Improvement made, the caregiver moves on.
But caregiving for someone with Alzheimer's
Holds no such promise. The most one can hope for
Is a holding pattern, and even that is limited in duration,
And before long caregiving has taken on a life of its own:
Days fade into months and months go by
Like the pages of a book, caregiving becomes the norm,
Past life barely remembered as the one being cared for fades,
Less and less able to do for himself,
And the caregiver, picking up the slack,
Fades from her former self—
Two people lost to one disease.

Letting Go

Letting go is one of my least favorite things to do.
You have only to look in my closet to understand.
By nature I am deeply sentimental,
Attached to houses, people, places visited.
I have never been good at good-bye,
Preferring to slip out the door unnoticed,
But now I am faced with letting go
Of my husband,
Our former life,
Our hopes and dreams,
Piece by piece
Day by day
Year by year,
Of old resentments,
Unfinished business,
Expectations never met
That no longer serve us,
Cannot be resolved,
Belong to another time and place,
And the by-product of letting go
Is the space it creates for change
As I adapt to this man who is my husband,

Just not the one I married,
As I reconstruct my life,
That had become comfortable and predictable,
To something that will support me now and in the future,
As I adjust my hopes and dreams,
At a time when they were just coming true,
To something more realistic, more workable.
And I know it is a process,
Not a linear path to be followed
But instead to be worked through
In one's own time and way.
Still, a part of me wants to close my eyes,
Hold on to everything I've known and loved,
While another part of me waits expectantly in the wings
To witness the metamorphosis.

Tips: The Caregiver's Lexicon

BA: life Before Alzheimer's, **AA:** life After Alzheimer's.

Absentee: a friend or relative who doesn't know what to say or do, so stays away or hides out in produce when they see you in the grocery store.

Bad Karma: what the "enlightened" tell you is the reason why someone gets Alzheimer's, and why caregiving is your intended purpose/fate in life.

Boundaries: the parameters that caregivers set concerning what they can and cannot do. An essential tool if the caregiver doesn't want to face burnout or illness brought on by exhaustion and overload.

Breakthrough: also known as an "epiphany," when one sees the situation as it is, not as one would like it to be; sometimes can be years coming.

Buffer Zone: a necessary distance between person cared for and caregiver.

Caregiver Dementia: a condition that presents itself as dementia, but is a temporary condition brought on by overload. Rx: Happy pills or respite.

Caregiver Meltdown: when the caregiver is overwhelmed and looses it. Exhibited behavior has much in common with the terrible two's, except they pull it off.

Caregiver Sanity Check: "Your loved is doing well or is fine or same as before."

Compassion Fatigue: the inability over the long term to sustain the commitment and fulfillment of the beginning stage.

Confabulation: stories told with little accuracy or truth to them.

Defining moment: a moment that can't be ignored, often bringing change.

Drive-by visits: friends, family, relatives stop by for a visit that is over before it begins.

Flicker of the light bulb: those brief moments when person returns to former self.

Gifts of Love: little white lies that all caregivers tell.

Good Intentions: what others purport they had when nothing is done.

Great Expectations: a set of unrealistic, wishful expectations that caregivers often hold about their role, how things should go, and what others should do.

Lost & Found: a common condition where an item can be missing for hours, days, weeks, months, only to suddenly reappear.

Married widow/widower: unofficial matrimonial status of spousal caregivers.

Martyr: what a caregiver can quickly become if not careful. Important to remember that martyrs are only rewarded and revered after their death.

No Man's Land: a place where those dealing with dementia reside.

Normal: there is *real normal*, what is happening out in the world, and *caregiver normal*, which is the adjustment one made to the situation, rendering it the *new normal*.

Out of Sync: how the caregiver feels in comparison to the rest of the world.

Poltergeist: often the one blamed for missing items, because everyone knows you cannot argue or blame a person with dementia.

Respite: touted by all as the antidote to caregiver stress, but is in truth more of a dream than a reality.

Reentry: what happens when the caregiver returns from a respite.

Sainthood: what the public likes to make caregivers into.

Second childhood: what people with dementia get to experience again.

Second time around: not referring to marriage, but to being a parent again.

Shadow: a 24-7 companion you are never without, your new best friend.

Survivor: what all caregivers hope to be at the conclusion. Not to be confused with the TV show, which is amateurish in comparison.

Survivor tools: black humor and fantasy.

Underrated: the contribution that caregivers and families make.

"We really must get together, I'll call you": an exit line used by the faint of heart.

Window of Opportunity: amount of quality time still left.

Transition

How do you know if the person you are caring for has transitioned from beginning stage into middle stage? While much has been written on the subject, clinical behaviors documented, timelines given, score indicators on the mini-mental exam outlined, the best indication is the caregiver's behavior and perception of the situation. While no one wants to see or admit to the progression of the illness, by middle stage, denial is no longer an option nor has it any value.

I held on to the beginning stage as long as I could. I would actually hold my breath and pray while my husband took the mini-mental, as if I had magic powers that would make the disease stop dead in its tracks. It was only with the heightening of his existing behaviors, along with the introduction of some new behaviors on both our parts, that I was able to admit to myself that he had entered the middle stage. One of the best indicators was the greater decline of his functional abilities.

His increased slowness is probably what frustrated me the most, and often led to my anger. Intellectually, I knew the truth of the saying "You can never hurry an Alzheimer's patient," but living it was something else. It gives a whole new meaning to the word "slow." Grocery shopping became a half-day event, I lost him in the rush of Grand Central Terminal, getting him out of the house was a major undertaking, and time seemed to slow almost to a halt. My life was now completely taken up with him, with very little time left over for me—another indicator that middle stage had arrived.

Finally, one day it happened: my frustration got the best of me. We discovered that he had lost his credit card ("preserving dignity") as we were on the way out the door to the airport. I had to stop, call the credit card company, and then put them on hold while he got my purse, a task that proved to be too much for him and me both. In a torrent of frustration, I simultaneously attacked him verbally and with my fist. It was a perfectly horrifying moment for me, and while I do not condone my behavior, for the first time, I was able to understand the genesis of such behavior. There is no excuse for it, and the best I can offer is that it was not planned and came out of nowhere. This is what I have come to call a "defining moment," and it was this moment that cemented my decision to get help and to try to get my life back in order. Much is written about having patience and not blaming the person who has the disease. Ninety-nine percent of the time this makes sense; it is in the one percent where the danger lies. Until you have taken care of someone with ongoing decline for many years, you will not know how precariously close a caregiver can come to the edge. When I discussed this with my psychologist in a session, I said, "Well, at least he won't remember it." To which he replied, "But you will." Truer words were never spoken. It will always stand out in my mind as one of my darkest moments.

Most caregivers are unprepared for the range and intensity of the emotional challenges of caregiving. Caregiving is a continual process of adjustment to stress and loss. While one can call on many defenses—denial, anesthetization of feelings, distancing—in the end, the only way through is to grieve. And caregivers do this each and every day by letting go of the dreams and expectations, and accepting the sadness, anger, frustration, and loss. The grieving process necessitates acknowledging painful emotions that defy predictability and control, but doing so opens caregivers to a new way of dealing with the situation.

As the tediousness of my days increased, along with the physical and mental exhaustion, I finally took the plunge, fortunate enough to be able to afford to hire a part-time companion and use supplemental daycare services. I had to juggle and figure out how to budget outside caregiving and support. There are many ways of reaching out to outside resources that can help support you. The first step is to contact the local Alzheimer's Association, and your town government, about what services are available for caregivers. As I worked at finding resources for my husband, I was also looking for ways to supplement my income, having given up a lucrative career. I knew I couldn't work full time again, but I needed the income and the mental and interpersonal stimulation that went along with a job. After much research and unwillingness to give up, I was able to meet both our needs.

As I look back on it, I wish I had arranged for outside help sooner. Part of me felt I could and should do it myself, while the other part didn't want to acknowledge my husband's transition into middle stage. I wasted precious time and caused unnecessary damage to us both. It's common knowledge that caregivers wait too long to get help. In the beginning, I couldn't understand how this could occur. Now I know. I only hope that when the next stage arrives, I won't make the same mistake. I'd like to say middle stage got easier as it went along and I adjusted, but it's not that simple. Some aspects of that statement are true, but my heightened awareness of the devastation of this horrific disease made it almost unbearable. Nothing in life prepares one for this—nothing.

New Role

I have added a new role
One I barely noticed
Sliding into it on automatic pilot
Lulled by his holding pattern
His mini-mental state remaining the same
Unchanged from a year ago,
But I have suddenly become the director of his day
In much greater detail.
Gone is the simple three-objective list for the day,
Replaced by explicit step-by-step directions.
Everything must be spelled out,
Explained once and then again.
Coming very subtly,
Registering as overload one day,
He needs more supervision.
I, the caregiver, am the gauge,
The internal instrument by which no behavior
Passes unnoticed.

Slipped

He has slipped.
There is more confusion,
Evidence that he understands less and less,
Favorite activities forgotten
As if they never existed.
He no longer drives,
Nor is able to find some rooms or certain objects
In the house,
And he cannot be left alone.
He has slipped, but so have I.
My world is made up of exhaustion,
Defined by tasks and chores, elementary in nature.
No time for my activities,
Running on borrowed time
Consumed by the needs of his world.

Domino Effect

He is losing ground.
Things once familiar are fading to a distant background
Or to not at all.
He needs more assistance with activities of daily living,
No longer can be left alone.
But I too am losing ground
Overwhelmed by increasing responsibilities
Less time for self,
Increasingly forgetful and accident prone,
Like a domino effect we exist in reaction to his disease.

He's Gone

"He's gone."
That is what the neurologist said to me during our last visit.
"He's gone."
I find myself referring to him as "that man" in my mind.
After all, he is no longer the man I married
He's become "that man."
I tell the doctor he still presents well,
And he replies, " A pianist can still play,
Even if it's only one tune."
My son on a recent visit home exclaims,
"Dad is just a shell of himself."
And I am careful not to add, "A shattered shell,"
My son's grief far too apparent.
He's gone.
A unanimous decision on all our parts,
But where has he gone?

Shell

"Dad is just a shell of himself," my son tells me
During a recent visit,
Having not seen him in months.
I feel the words forming as my defenses take hold:
"We can still have conversations, enjoy movies,
Go to dinner, limited as it may be, we can still do this,"
But I remain silent,
Transfixed by the sadness on my son's face.
I am losing a husband far too early
I know what that feels like.
He is losing his father long before a son should;
I cannot imagine that pain.
I am desperately holding onto any semblance of normality,
He is struggling to come to terms with an unbearable reality.
Through his eyes I see what it is I have not wanted to see.
Now, I wonder what it is he sees through my eyes?

Lost It

He has lost his wallet with his credit card in it,
Coming at the most inopportune time
With no time to spare.
My fault for still letting him carry one,
"Preserving his dignity" has gone too far.
I am frantically on the phone with the credit card company,
While he retrieves my purse so I can match numbers.
Minutes pass, mounting one by one,
He has not returned from this simple errand.
Putting the credit card company on hold,
I go to look for him,
Find him standing in the kitchen looking lost,
My purse two feet away.
"You can't do the simplest thing." I shout at him,
As my hand simultaneously hauls off and socks him.
I am frozen in my tracks,
Startled by what has occurred,
Startled by my actions,
But not so startled as the look upon his face.

Next Time

I hit him.
I don't know who was more surprised,
Shock registering on his otherwise blank face,
Horror filling up inside of me. I hit him
In anger, in frustration, out of exhaustion,
All reasons why, none valid.
I am well educated, middle class,
Versed in the complexities of this disease
And still I hit him. I could not stop myself… out of control,
Swinging at him as my rage reached its crescendo,
Shouting "Can't you do anything right?"
What did I expect, an answer, an apology?
That should come from me, not him.
I am wrong and I know it, but what I fear most is
Will there be a next time?

Door

I kicked the door in a moment of rage, leaving a crack.
The same door my son, at fifteen, put his fist through
In a moment of rage, leaving a gaping indentation.
I was shocked when he did that,
Wondering where that level of rage came from,
Fearing his anger and the depth of this emotions.
Now I understand.

Point of No Return

I have reached it… the point of no return.
We can not go on living like this, but I am not ready
To let him go, put him in assisted living
As some have suggested or politely hinted at.
It is not time, I am not ready yet,
But we cannot go on like this.
It is time to hire a companion, find daycare
And change the structure of our life.
I have become the caregiver I read about in the books,
Waiting too long, unable to do what must be done,
Something I thought I would never be, not understanding it
When I read about it, not understanding it even now,
Except in the context of the power
Of the hold on me to keep things as normal as I can
For as long as I can. But look at the price.

Props

They lie around the house… props. His wallet,
Devoid of any importance, newspapers partially read
But not to be thrown out, stock quotes blasting continually
On the finance channel, financial magazines begging
To be read. Sometimes I want to throw these props out
Stop pretending our life is normal, but I don't and I won't
I can't. These props support the second act—middle stage.

Tips on Transition

Must Reads:

Boss, Pauline, *Ambiguous Loss*. Harvard University Press, Cambridge, Mass.

Shenk, David. *The Forgetting*. Doubleday, New York.

Viorst, Judith. *Necessary Losses*. Simon and Schuster, New York.

Accepting Life as It Is

God, grant me the serenity
To accept the things I cannot change
The courage to change the things I can,
And the wisdom to know the difference.

Exercises for Positive Change

"Heavy Load No More" Exercise

1. On a sheet of paper, draw a rock; inside of it list one thing or person you are now trying to control.
2. Continue to draw rocks until you have listed everything.
3. When finished, observe how large is the pile you have been carrying around with you. Let yourself feel the weight.
4. Now decide what you can control or be responsible for and what is out of your control.
5. Cross off those things that are out of your control.
6. Now start the conscious process of letting go of them.

"Worry" Exercise

1. Draw five columns.
2. Label column one "Worry Column," and list everything you have worried about in the past few months.
3. In column two, put a check mark next to those things that turned out all right.
4. In column three, put a check mark next to the items that benefited from your worry.
5. In column four, evaluate what worry has accomplished both positively and negatively for you.
6. In column five, surrender those things for which worry has no benefit.
7. Now, with what is left, make an *action plan* for things you can change.

Impact

As I wrestled with the impact of our transition into middle stage and its many conflicting emotions, the hardest part was accepting the change in my attitude from hopeful to resigned. My goal had become survival for me and continued quality care for my husband. While the ultimate loss lay ahead, it was as if all the accumulated losses—ability to travel, companionship, a circle of friends to socialize with, a future—became the practice ground. Day by day our former life slipped away, until it seemed only my husband remembered it. Often throughout the years, various doctors and members of my support group told me that, as my husband progressed, we would become work, and friends would start to dwindle. Unfortunately, as we moved more into middle stage, this dire prediction came true.

During this period I started to take on some new behaviors. I became a major klutz, often tripping over my own feet, having minor car accidents and trips to the emergency room. One person living a life for two is overwhelming. A turning point came when I received my second traffic ticket in the same month—this time for going through a red light. This signaled to me what I refer to as a "defining moment." Such moments seem to come out of nowhere, when in actuality they have been occurring regularly, but we have chosen to ignore them. What finally makes it a "defining moment" is the fact that it can no longer be ignored. The red light incident forced me to look at what was happening, and I knew then that I had to begin to define boundaries if I was to survive.

As I took on new behaviors, so did my husband. Some were very strange, such as his need to eat only one food group at a time, not being able to see what was in front of him, often getting into the back seat of the car, and sometimes ending up on the floor in the middle of the night. A good sense of humor and a support group to share these things with is very helpful.

In one of our most endearing moments, my husband, wearing his lobster boxer shorts as bottoms, walked the dog. My family was appalled when I told them the story, but I found his newfound freedom refreshing and long overdue. Some of his new behaviors became a benefit to me and helped make my job easier. He seemed to forget about many things that were once important to him, resulting in a reduction of our magazine subscriptions and newspapers to a more workable number. He no longer cared if I entered his den, and the binders on his shelf and the contents of his desk drawer, once off limits, no longer were. Sadly, what I discovered was stacks and stacks of clippings from various newspapers, and articles from what seemed like year one. Middle stage afforded me the opportunity to clean house and get things more organized. I became a fan of the minimalist approach and today our house is simplified, which makes for less confusion and easier retrieval of missing items (not all!). I learned to use this approach in my own life to focus on only the truly important.

It is painful to face one's limitations, one's less-than-generous thoughts and feelings, but it's also liberating. I found myself being more direct with family instead of wrapping my husband's condition and my emotions in saccharine messages. It also became a time when I wrestled with the messages I had received while growing up, about what it meant to be a woman. Often, I felt in conflict with the dark, or shadow, side of myself. At first I was repulsed, but as I began to let this side of me emerge and not hide from it, I began to appreciate certain aspects, and integrate them into my personality. I was more than happy to begin saying good-bye to "the pleaser," the good-girl role I had played all my life. This is an ongoing process, with more to let go of and more to embrace, and while I have far to go, I now feel whole. Along with these changes, I have felt a shift to becoming more "spiritual."

The emotions of sadness, loss, and loneliness are predominant when I think of middle stage. One moment, my heart felt deep sadness, and the next moment it became hardened. I swung back and forth between emotions, partly out of self-protection and partly out of not knowing how to hold two conflicting emotions at the same time. It's been a struggle to learn how, and I often wished there were some formula I could apply. But the truth is, learning to sit with your emotions, allowing yourself to feel them and becoming comfortable with them is all that's needed. The loss that all caregivers feel is unlike any other. It is a gradual loss, in which the essence of the person, and all the trappings you knew and loved, fade away. For me, letting go has been a difficult process of continually mourning each loss as its occurs. As the losses and the loneliness increase, I've been forced more and more to construct a strong inner world where I can connect with myself and find sustenance. While our inner world is always available to us, caregivers must also make sure to reach out to the outer world. New friendships with people in the same or similar situation are just waiting to be made and a source of great comfort. And don't forget about pets—our dog is a wonderful companion to both of us, and brings laughter to the house with his antics. He serves a dual role: first as a companion to my husband, then as a buffer zone that leaves me feeling less smothered.

What amazes me most is that, even in the midst of all of this, there still are moments of joy and beauty. Perhaps it is loss that compels us to look with reverence at the everyday happenings and begin to see with new eyes. I miss our old life, and would give anything to have it back, with one exception—I would like to bring the new me along.

The New Me

The new me is alive and kicking,
Not so different from the old.
After all, we each have a core from which we operate,
But the new me puts up with less,
Cuts to the point quicker,
Understands and applies the meaning of choice,
Is not driven by duty unless it is duty defined by me.
The new me has a softness,
An appreciation of the plight of others,
A respect for the trials and tribulations of life.
The new me is less judgmental of others and self,
Content to let people be who they are,
But careful not to get tangled up where I don't belong
Or in that which does not serve me.
The new me understands that selfish is not always bad,
And that I have needs that also must be addressed and met.
The new me has cleaned closets both real and metaphorical,
Learned to travel lighter,
Appreciate the moment,
And feel gratitude for the good in my life,
But what a long time coming
And such a high price to pay.

Defining Moments

There are defining moments in the course of this disease,
Moments that forever alter the course of the journey,
Different in nature and degree from other moments,
Crying out to be heard, refusing to be ignored.
In the beginning stage,
When denial becomes no longer an option,
And ones knows with certainty
That something is terribly wrong,
The defining moment forces us to face what was previously
Too painful to acknowledge, and cements the truth forever.
But in the middle stage, the moments are subtler in nature,
Harder to ascertain,
Having grown used to the craziness of this existence,
Where much is now taken for granted and accepted,
And a peace, a new way of being acclimatized,
Until suddenly,
One of these defining moments returns to take hold,
Grabs the attention of the caregiver and screams,
"I am back, pay attention!"
And in that moment the caregiver is yanked
From a life grown accustomed to,
And thrust without choice into middle stage,
And like all defining moments, different for each of us,
Propels us to where we need to go,
The next stop on our journey.

Martha Stewart

In the beginning I wanted to be "the perfect caregiver,"
A Martha Stewart of sorts
(before the stock market debacle).
Heaven knows why, I never really admired her,
But somehow it seemed appropriate in my new role
And the hidden agenda was, "I can beat this disease."
In the beginning it seemed possible
And I often wondered what the fuss was about—
A few misplaced objects,
A lost item here or there,
A mess in the kitchen,
Clothes all over the floor,
All in a day's work.
That was then, surpassed by now
Increasing confusion,
Growing dependencies,
Mounting responsibilities,
And a level of fatigue I've never known before.
Five-plus official years* into the disease,
Martha Stewart holds no interest,
Her name banned from my vocabulary
Along with the concept of perfect,
For now I know just getting through the day is enough,
My hidden agenda long gone.
I can't beat this disease;
I just pray it won't beat me.

* *From point of diagnosis*

Lost Voice

The story is the same, only the storyteller changes.
I've heard it countless times before,
From the support group leader,
From the assisted living coordinator of the dementia unit,
From fellow caregivers,
From an audience member eager to share her story.
They speak of the tears that flow
Out of nowhere without warning,
Greater in magnitude
Different than before,
Tears that would not cease
Until hospitalization or medication,
Until someone stepped in and proclaimed,
"We cannot lose two people to this disease."
Something the storyteller knew all along
But was powerless to articulate.

Long Hours

The worst time is at night
After sleep has run its course
And the long, dark hours loom ahead,
When nothing looks bright
And the world is full of monsters
And one wonders if daylight will come.
It is in those hours while the rest of the world sleeps
That the caregiver lies awake
Feeling alone, fearing for the future
Worrying about the present,
Knowing that sleep is a requirement
to make it through the day,
But the whirling, churning mind pays no heed
Preferring to stay stuck on red alert.
There is no peace, no respite
This disease is 24-7.

Survivor

I watched "Survivor," along with forty million Americans,
Fascinated, held hostage each week to the television,
Asking myself, "Why?"
Realizing that in some strange way, unconscious till now,
I related to being on an island, cut off from the real world,
The mission just to survive.

Seasons

We are living in a season of hell
The death march moving on,
Leaving in its wake confusion and a shadow of a former self
Nothing on the horizon to hold out hope.
The days have become one like another
Begging the question, "Is this any way to live?"
We are living in a season of plenitude
And upcoming marriage,
One grandchild full of life, another newly welcomed,
Bringing some relief and partial answer to the question,
"Is this any way to live?"
One season a curse
The other a blessing
Reminding me that life is a complex balance.

Vacation

I pack his bag, drive him to the airport,
Park the car, lug the bags and check us in,
Assist him through the metal detector,
Direct him to his seat, strapping him in tight,
Unpack his newspaper, oversee his food,
Collect our baggage, find the way to the hotel,
Check us both in, unpack his clothes,
Sit by him on the beach as he sleeps,
Make conversation for two as we eat.
This is my vacation too, although it does not feel that way.
Once they were getaways, vacations for two,
Retreats from the world. Now we bring our world with us.

Brief Moment

I skip over the stones, adeptly dodging the incoming tide
Caught up in a world of my own, unaware he is behind me
Until I turn around and see him stranded, not knowing
Which way to turn, not knowing what to do next
Looking helpless and confused. It is painful to witness,
Highlighting how compromised his world has become,
Magnifying his deficits.
For a brief moment
I had forgotten the truth that guides our life.
It is those moments that keep me sane.

Option

I stand on the precipice barely aware of the jagged coral
Underneath my feet. Far below the azure waters wait
Tranquil, in spite of a 400-foot waterfall
Cascading downward.
Straight ahead the lure of freedom calls,
An option suddenly appears.
Only a few short steps and the descent begins
Mine, not his, and I contemplate for a brief moment
How easy it would be. Who would know?
They would assume I slipped
Or simply misjudged.

Sunglasses

The salesman at the beach cabana
Tall, blonde and handsome, the ultimate Maui god,
Tries to interest me in a pair of sunglasses,
Looking with obvious disdain at my grocery store special
As he drones on and on expounding the virtues
Of the glasses: Endorsed by the U.S. Ski Team
Indestructible to the elements,
Unaware his rhetoric is not reaching me,
That there is no connection
Until he mentions the world appears rose colored
And I perk up and lay my MasterCard down.

Frozen Solid

Alone on a rock by the edge of the ocean, I sit
Basking in the warmth of the sun, so different
From the cold back home. The sky a remarkable blue
Playing off the ocean, an array of ever-changing hues,
In contrast to the gray of East Coast winters,
The warmth of the sun, the sound of the waves
Lulling me into a state of semi-consciousness.
No longer alert, in control—a luxury unknown to me—
I feel myself beginning to thaw out from the continual long
Winter that has become the landscape of my life.
Still, no matter how intense the heat, how beckoning the sun,
There remains a small, impenetrable part of me frozen solid.

Vacation

The Mexican coastline where the Aztec Ocean
Meets the desert, is breathtaking. The ocean
A remarkable blue, playing off the ambient breezes,
The hotel exquisite, mariachi music, abundant tropical
Foliage, a friendly waitstaff, eager to please,
Create the ambiance. It is a dream vacation
As evidenced by the guests busy with endless activities
Or simply lolling by the pool, putting their other lives aside.
My husband eats in great abundance, sleeps at every
Opportunity, and follows right behind me wherever I go.
We do not have the luxury of putting our life aside—
It follows us wherever we go.

Vacation for One

We are on vacation
The villa is lovely, the ocean magnificent
The atmosphere romantic
A picture-perfect vacation marred only by the truth.
We are in direct contrast to the other guests
Alone in our home I have adapted.
Out in the world I am forced to face the truth,
It is a vacation for one.

Differentiation

I am alone, something I have known for some time.
I am lonely, something I have known only recently.
Alone and lonely, not the same,
A distinction needing to be made,
But first both must be admitted to.
Why did it take me so long to admit I was lonely?
Was I trying so hard to hold it all together,
Or was it simply being on vacation
Surrounded by other couples
That forced me to admit to myself I am lonely?
I am alone even when I am next to him.
I can live with that.
I am lonely.
That is much harder to live with.

Just Happened

I have stopped writing, promising myself I would
Carve out a moment here and there, but it never came.
My life is full of his needs, a day planned around his schedule,
And when a quiet moment comes
I am too drained to do anything but sit.
I have lost myself to this disease in my role of caregiver.
Not planning to, it just happened unnoticed
As I quietly took over more and more of his life
And had less and less of my own.
Without knowing, I became a prisoner,
My writing, which was my therapy, simply ceased.
My job, which was my identity, given up
So I could spend the time we had left together
My friends, whom I shared much with,
No longer held the same commonality.
My world shrunk, and in doing so
Became easier and more manageable,
No longer forced to make communication for two
Or cover for him in public so we appear just another couple,
Or fight the rigors of travel, finding it easier to stay home.
None of this a conscious decision, it just happened
Out of weariness, exhaustion, depleted resources.
But now I must find my way out of this narrow existence
Before it becomes too comfortable
And I too am lost.

Fantasy

He is angry with me:
He did not get his way,
Having grown used to getting his way.
I am angry with him.
We are locked in a power struggle
Simplistic in nature, but still a power struggle.
He plays his trump card, throwing his glasses on the floor.
I want to step on them, crush them,
I see it played out before me,
I can even feel my anger drain out of me so vivid is it.
But reality beckons me back,
I would only be left to pick up the pieces,
The one responsible for replacing the glasses,
So I walk away, satisfied instead with my fantasy.

Morphed

I blew two tires on the SUV while running errands,
Rounded the exit, not seeing the black ice,
And smashing the side of the jeep into the guardrail,
Ended up in the emergency room after cutting my hand,
Spent endless hours looking for items I have misplaced,
Been treated for high blood pressure, eczema, and stress,
Made numerous simple errors at work,
Forgotten which exit to take off the highway,
Made decisions I later regretted simply to be free of them,
Watched as dishes slipped from my hands,
Smashing into tiny pieces,
Sent letters out without stamps, paid bills twice or not at all,
Racked up enough late payments that I wished
They were frequent flyer miles,
Forgotten to give him his medicine or take mine,
Hit my head on the fireplace, ending up with a concussion.
I've morphed into someone I no longer recognize.
He may have the illness
But I carry the symptoms.

Slow Down

"Slow down, you move too fast,"
Lyrics of an old song run through my head
Reminding me I need to slow down,
But in a world of cell phones, emails,
constant communication, and a type-A personality,
It is almost impossible.
I can survive the same question asked over and over,
The tediousness of the same remarks that comprise our day,
The shadowing of my every move,
His inability to do for himself.
But the slowness of his world
A snail's pace at best,
His life almost at a standstill
Is driving me crazy.
We have become the tortoise and the hare.

Meltdowns

Like an alien force, an evil spirit coming over me,
One day something snapped,
Meltdowns became my escape,
Making me feel like I was teetering on the brink,
No longer capable of handling the situation.
The doctor became increasingly concerned.
I did not want happy pills
Nor did I want blood pressure pills.
I wanted my life back,
The one this disease had taken away,
Along with the declining stock market
Limiting my options, cementing my fate.
Then I discovered the gym,
Something I previously had no interest in,
Now it is my haven, my refuge,
Where I go to exorcise my demons.

Meltdown Day

He has removed all the items I loaded into the Jeep
For the dump, returning them to the garage.
He took the directions for the vacuum cleaner
That took me two hours to put together,
Returning them to God only knows where.
He has misplaced his watch, on which he cannot tell time,
And wants me to join him on his search—fat chance.
It is not a good day. My patience is gone.
Perhaps I will find it in the place where he put
The vacuum directions and all will be well again.
It is too late, I have a meltdown letting loose
With a banshee-like scream. It feels so good, so freeing,
I wonder did the neighbors hear? It is too late to care.
My pride, my dignity long gone. I have become just like
Meltdown Maddie, my granddaughter,
Both of us delighting in the terrible twos!

Context

Today was a bad day. I yelled, lost my temper,
Had a major meltdown, said things of which I am ashamed,
But at the moment felt justified. Alone, with all the
Responsibilities this illness brings, hateful, resentful feelings
Get stirred up. I find myself repelled by the person
I have become. I could beat myself up, wallow in despair,
feel even worse than I do now. But I choose, instead,
To put it in context. Today was a bad day.

Shattered

I watch as one of a pair of our favorite champagne glasses,
Solely designated for celebrations,
Slips from my hand. I try to break the fall
But to no avail; there is nothing I can do.
Much like the sensation of an impending traffic accident
My eyes follow the glass until it hits bottom.
Our favorite set, holding years of collected memories,
Happy events, celebrations,
Shattered, leaving one glass alone
Like I now am.

Fantasy

My fantasy has returned
The one about being rescued from this nightmare
The one about awakening to find it only a bad dream.
I no longer believe in this fantasy
Nor cling to the hope it will come true
Although at times I still indulge myself,
Enjoying the brief respite.
But now with more experience under my belt
I use this fantasy for what it is—
An indicator that I have reached my breaking point,
I am working on reserves.

Change of Heart

I used to be judgmental, full of pronouncements,
Before the illness.
Case in point: my mother's friend,
The second wife who could no longer care for her husband
Who developed Alzheimer's five years into the marriage.
In my infinite wisdom,
I concluded her behavior was typical second-wife syndrome.
I listened to women in my support group,
Whose husbands were further along than mine,
Elaborate on how they could no longer
Tolerate the mess or the strain,
And in my infinite wisdom, I thought, what's the big deal?
I used to think self-sacrifice was what marriage was about,
So my career, my life, took back stage
Despite it being the era of consciousness raising,
And in my infinite wisdom, dismissed the message.
I used to think being female made me responsible
For everyone and everything
A belief indoctrinated from the moment of birth,
And in my infinite wisdom,
Being the good girl, I dared not question it.
I used to give literal interpretation to the vow,
"In sickness and in health"
Even if the cost meant my health, too,
So, in my infinite wisdom,
I vowed no spouse of mine would go into a nursing home.

I would like to think I have grown wiser with the years
But the plain truth is, I have grown wiser with the disease.
No longer will I assume responsibility
For everyone and everything
Or judge others whose course or choices
Are different than mine
Or sacrifice my health and sanity—
The price is too high.
There are two people in this equation
And the illness tips the scales so drastically
That if I am to survive, if I want to be of any service to him,
I have to give up my judgments,
Lay my infinite wisdom aside,
And open myself to new ways of being.

Quality of Life

How can there be quality of life
For someone afflicted with Alzheimer's?
Is the term not an oxymoron
When one has been robbed of the most precious gift,
When days are locked into an endless repetition
Of questions and phrases,
Years mirror one another
And the progression continues its slow steady decline?
How can there be quality of life
For the caregiver
When the caregiving hours increase
With the progression of the disease,
The home is turned into a fortress,
And the caregiver becomes a prisoner
With burnout the inevitable conclusion?
Those were questions I wrestled with
When first faced with the impact of this disease
Questions that mirrored my feelings and beliefs.
But over the years I have had to challenge
My responses to these questions
Come to terms with my conflicting feelings
Factor into the equation the needs of both parties
And redefine the definition of quality of life,
And I have come to understand
That there will come a time for me to let go
To place my husband in a different environment

Where his functional abilities are maximized
And his independence promoted
Where he will have options and his dignity will be preserved
So setting a table becomes a source of pride, not a chore
Waving his arms and legs in group dance
Not silly but meaningful
Lingering over memories of the past,
Simply not a way to pass time but an occasion
And I will need to remind myself at those moments
That quality, like beauty, is in the eye of the beholder
And if I can let go of what was, accept my new role,
Work through the accompanying sadness and loss,
Be secure in the knowledge I have done all I could,
Then I believe peace will follow
Bringing with it a new definition of quality
In a life forever changed.

Amazed

Sometimes I am amazed at the beauty of the sunset,
The laughter we still can share,
The silliness over something the dog has done,
The delight in the antics of our grandchildren,
Amazed that in the darkness of this illness
There can still be these moments.
In spite of it all,
Life still shines through.

Tips Tried And True

Bed and Bath

- A long, narrow bed pillow to place between the two of you
- California Closets concept that can be purchased for much less at Home Depot. Organizes clothing; this is one of the best decisions I ever made and has made my life much easier.
- Colored his-and-her bath towels (two different colors)
- Labeled clothes drawers
- Rainforest shower head, very gentle and non-threatening; also, a bench to sit on
- Blue-colored tidy bowl cleaner
- Wall behind toilet painted a dark contrasting color
- Nightlights and flashlights
- Baby gate at top and bottom of stairs
- Sleeping problems: heartbeat teddy bear and/or sound machines that make a variety of noises
- Baby tearless shampoos and eye protectors

Kitchen

- Plastic dishes and glasses
- Dishes rearranged to lower shelf for easier access
- Cabinets labeled for contents
- Baby 1st locks for range and refrigerator, from K-mart type store or baby store
- Rubberized glass beach holders for glasses
- Answering service for telephone
- Caller ID so that all incoming calls are recorded
- Memory dialing phone
- Popsicles in freezer
- Medication dispensers

General

- Sound-and-light baby monitor so you don't have to be in the same room (Fisher Price)
- TV remote controller tied to table near couch or chair
- Ribbon on passenger front door or wherever they ride
- Electric dog fence: never worry again about Fido escaping
- Safe Return bracelets for both — a must
- Throwaway camera for special events
- Designated "crabby" T-shirt for caregiver, to let people know when you are at your wits' end
- Safety Plug-In's for electrical sockets
- Baby Bach tapes for evenings or for times of stress — very soothing and interesting to watch
- Large digital clock with day, time, and date
- Digital hand watch
- Eyeglasses that go from indoor to outdoors
- Bowl or basket by door for hat, gloves etc.
- Alarm system for house or door/window activated alarms (Radio Shack)
- Lost items finder (Radio Shack)
- Two-way radios (Radio Shack)
- Memory games
- Special hiding place for car keys

Out in the world

- Never leave home without it; wear it all the time and your wandering woes will be over: Safe Return Bracelet, (Safe Return, PO Box 9307, St. Louis, MO 63017-0307)
- At the movies sit in the back row where no will notice or care that he or she is asleep.

- When dining out, take an index card explaining the condition of the person for whom you are caring, and give it to the waiter.
- Play soothing music in the car and house.

Suggested Sources:

- Baby Store, Wal-Mart, K-mart
- Home Depot, Hardware store
- The Caregivers Marketplace (866/327-8340)
- The Alzheimer's Store (12633 159th Court, North Jupiter, Florida 33478)

Major Problem: My husband insisted on carrying a wallet with a credit card (I did convince him to go down to one card) in the house and when he went out with his companion. This is what is known as *preserving his dignity.* Often he would misplace it, which sent me into a tailspin because I was never sure if he had lost it while out with his companion or in the house.

Solution: I went to our local bank and took out a *debit card* in his name and put only a small amount of money in at any one time. I explained the situation to the bank, so only I can put more money into the account. He is now at the point where he has trouble signing his name, but the card goes with him everywhere.

Healthcare Professionals

Whenever I have a speaking engagement, during the question and answer period the topic invariably turns to healthcare professionals. It is a loaded subject that almost belongs with the *verboten* categories of religion and money, except audiences won't allow it. By the very nature of the disease, relationships that caregivers have with health care professionals are complex and long in duration. Since each caregiver brings their history with them, I can only speak from my vantage point. I have a great deal of respect and appreciation for the doctors who are helping guide me along our journey, but at the same time I feel anger, disappointment, and occasionally, abandonment. In many ways it parallels or mirrors my conflicting feelings about the illness and my role.

Because there is so little that can be done during the middle stage, I find it very difficult, and visits to the neurologist seem to reflect this. It has become clear to me that most of what does not fall under the realm of clinical is met with a certain level of discomfort and resistance. Our neurologist, Jan Mashman, M.D., is a kind, deeply caring physician who, like all doctors today, is under strict time guidelines dictated by insurance companies. I have the feeling that many doctors are dancing as fast as they can, and many patients are missing the old days when there was time to ask questions and voice concerns. It took me a long time to understand and accept this and seek help in the appropriate place.

Naively, I expected our neurologist to be all things to caregivers (me), often causing tension, I'm sure, in both of us. I will be forever grateful for the words he gave me upon diagnosis. Drawing one of his infamous charts designed to depict where I presently was and where I would be at the end, he threw me a lifeline: "You will come through this and be okay." I am confident that he will be there at the end where he has more of a role; it is this middle stage I am struggling through alone.

Our primary doctor, Warren Cohn, M.D., has been a source of comfort to both of us. When I want to stop taking a certain medicine, he reminds me of how long the journey is and of the different kinds of help needed. When I am frightened about who will take care of me if I become very ill, he listens and lets me know he will be there. He is unique to the profession and I feel blessed to have him. Wonderful listener though he is, I've still on occasion had to hit him over the head with a point. He is not an Alzheimer's specialist and, like all doctors, is trained to extend lives. We spent some time arguing over a colonoscopy for my husband before he was able to hear and respect my wishes.

It is my psychologist, Stephen Eliot, Ph.D., to whom I went immediately after receiving the official diagnosis and to whom I credit much of my coping abilities. I sat in a stupor, surrounded by an incredible feeling of comfort and the knowledge that I would not be alone on this journey, while alternately feeling paralyzed by fear and terror. It is here that I can face my fears, ugly thoughts, and raw emotions; construct the needed personal boundaries; gain the strength to put aside the many opinions of others and listen to my own voice, and begin the process of preparing for a new life, while simultaneously dealing with what life has dealt. Here I am not alone with the terrors and demands of this hideous disease.

Carl Rotenberg, M.D., in conjunction with my psychologist and internist, oversees the medication I need to help make the journey easier. I appreciate his respect of my wishes to not be overmedicated, and his kind, gentle manner.

Even having this cadre of doctors, I felt a lingering sense of frustration and wanted someone who was a guru in both the clinical and emotional aspects of the disease. Through a friend I found Malcolm Gordon, M.D., a semi-retired psychiatrist with a specialty in Alzheimer's. In his office I was able to learn about the intricacies of the disease, explore behaviors (both my husband's and mine), and have my questions welcomed and dealt with. I didn't feel like an irritant, nor did I have I have to go to great lengths for him to get the picture. Most amazing is his uncanny sense of timing. During one visit, he wanted to explore the issue of losing my husband, despite my assurances that it was not presently a problem; the very next week I lost him in Grand Central Terminal. Dr. Gordon is always a step ahead of me, preparing me for what is to come. With his keen understanding of the effects on both patient and caregiver, I use our occasional time together to help both my husband and myself.

Finally, I would be remiss if I did not mention the leader of my women's support group and of my husband's group. Roni Lang, MSW, director of the Stamford Geriatric Assessment Center, brings a clear understanding of the disease process, along with constant support and abundant kindness. Her willingness to give of her time to help caregivers see their needs as legitimate has been of great benefit to all of us.

The healthcare professionals we have dealt with have been understanding and supportive. I have tried to respect their time and come to each visit with a list of questions, an outline of my husband's progress to date, and the knowledge that we are just one of many patients. It was not until the middle stage that I felt a sense of being in no man's land. Unlike the beginning stage, with its flurry of diagnosis and education, or the end stage, with its emphasis on palliative care and helping families deal with the inevitable, there is no agenda or protocol. Physicians become tightlipped about the future, visits are short, and support sorely lacking.

Documented research on caregiver burden shows a huge increase during the middle stage. Caregivers have wider concerns, while physicians are focused on treatment. Taking care of people with Alzheimer's has to be a partnership between physician and caregiver that covers management and treatment, as well as the other issues associated with caring for someone with the disease. While this would be so in an ideal or future state, I've come to realize that I expected too much from my neurologist, and was better off dealing with my emotional issues and needs with a therapist. Perhaps in the future there will be more integration of management and issues.

Thanks to a landmark decision made by the Bush administration in 2002, Medicare now includes treatment for Alzheimer's disease which includes mental health services, physical and occupational therapy, medications, hospice care, and care provided at home. Many of the strides that have been made in this arena are due to the hard work and diligence of those who advocate for the disease. Each spring, The Public Policy Forum is held in Washington, DC, where caregivers meet to learn more about the illness, are apprised of the latest research, and at the conclusion, spend a day calling on their congressional representatives. It is an amazing group of dedicated individuals who truly have impacted the direction of the support allocated for this disease. For more information on how to become a part of this group, contact your local Alzheimer's Association.

It's up to each of us as healthcare consumers to be vocal about our needs and to be prepared to go the second round. Many insurance companies bank on the hope that consumers will give up, thinking nothing can be done. Our healthcare system is a sad commentary on the richest, most productive nation in the world. It is even sadder that caregivers have to go the extra mile when dealing with an illness that already overtaxes their reserves.

No matter what my feelings are on any given day or situation, I am grateful for the healthcare professionals who have joined us on our journey.

Disconnect

Disconnect
It is the reason behind the helping professions'
need to educate the caregiver
Disconnect
When the synapses are covered with amyloids
Rendering them non-functioning
Disconnect
When families can't make the connection
Between strange behavior and dementia
Disconnect
When the patient is incapable of translating
The message into action
Disconnect
When caregiver emotions overcome the rational mind
Disconnect
When the helping profession has run out of options.

Advice*

"Just take him home and love him." That's how I know
My visit with the neurologist is coming to an end.
It is his sage advice dispensed at the close of each visit,
But what does it mean? There is no hope?
There is nothing more I can do?
And how does it apply to me?
Am I to be a courtesan or just the devoted wife?
Does it imply I am not seeing the big picture,
Grasping the situation in its entirety,
Or is it simply reality wrapped in nice words?
This is a terrible thing that should happen to no one.

Message

I did not understand the message from our neurologist
At the beginning: "Just take him home and love him."
I silently admonished him for being insensitive, chauvinistic
Not in touch with the reality of our situation
And, worse yet, medically wiping his hands clean.
Now years into the illness, I hear the message differently
And understand the context in which it was given
His hope that at the end I had no regrets,
And now with the clarity that time affords,
See the kindness behind it, not just for my husband,
But for me, the caregiver.

* From *Unplanned Journey: Understanding the Itinerary*, p. 61

Don't Get It

These damn doctors don't get it! Instead they offer
Solicitous words designed to soothe or perhaps
Just shut me up. I tell the psychologist how my husband
Lost his wallet, a prop to preserve his dignity,
And he couldn't understand my reaction,
Or, at least, the magnitude of it.
After all, it was just a matter of a few simple phone calls.
I guess he could see the disbelief on my face, for he went on
To explain how I should not feel responsible for everything.
My husband could call the credit card company,
Renew his driver's license now used for ID, and put in
For a new insurance card. Disbelief must still have been
Evident on my face, for he continued on,
That if it were his family, he would offer empathy,
Or perhaps even sympathy, but it would not be his problem,
Or, for that matter, much of a problem.
Perhaps he should watch as my husband struggles
With the electronic menu of choices, which drives
The rest of us to near-breakdown states, forgetting
The first choice as soon as the next has been offered.
And maybe if he spent a day in my shoes he would
Understand while it may be an occasional event in his family,
In mine it is the norm. And while I understand
His intentions are well meant, I hold fast to my belief,
Medical degrees aside, until you've lived it,
Experienced it on personal level, *you just don't get it!*

Face

"Don't give me that face, I can get that face at home,"
I shout at my therapist
Shocking us both or, at least, me.
"Where did that come from?" he asks me,
But I have no answer, only the feeling
I don't like his present face.
It is stern, without emotion, almost blank,
And while I know he is listening hard,
Thinking before he speaks, I do not like that face.
It reminds me of my husband's:
Stern, without emotion, blank.
I can deal with it at home—I have no choice,
But not in public.
I have seen him use that face before
It never bothered me until now
I am running on empty
Tired of living with someone who does not respond.
I cannot provoke a fight with my husband;
It will do no good,
But I can provoke a fight with my therapist.
It is a safe place to explore feelings
And so I transfer onto him the rage I feel at home,
Something he does not deserve.

Who's the Stupid One Here?

"He's stupid!"
That's what I tell my therapist.
Tired and fed up with my husband's ongoing behavior:
Not finding the correct car door, winding up in the back seat
Or worse yet, following right behind me to the driver's door,
Then standing there with his now infamous blank stare.
"He's not stupid," he replies. "He has Alzheimer's."
As if I forgot, as if it were something one could forget,
But it is and I did.
In my exhaustion, in my annoyance I confused the two
And reacted as if my husband were stupid.
Thank goodness I have my therapist to remind me,
To keep me on track when it is I who am being stupid.

My Therapist: Best Interest

I sit in my therapist's office
Unhappy with him for what I perceive as a minor offense,
Unhappy with myself in my response to him.
We try to iron it out, uncover issues
To no avail.
"It is in your best interest." he explains.
I leave feeling hurt
And for days his word toss around in my head,
Words and concepts unfamiliar to me.
Why wouldn't they be?
Used to putting other people's needs first
Never occurring to me that I could have a best interest
And if I could, certainly this disease has nullified it
Leaving me without choice, or am I?
Choices exist even when we cannot see them.
Perhaps, going forward I should take a page from his book
And consider what is in my best interest,
A point he has been driving home over the past months
Unsuccessfully, until now.

My Therapist: Luxury

I sit in my therapist's office
Far away from the demands of the disease
But the concerns sit right there next to me
Following along wherever I go.
His office is different:
Time slows down
It is tranquil no matter what is being discussed,
A haven of sorts.
The agenda belongs to me
The only time I have to truly focus on myself
Temporarily freed from watching over my husband,
Anticipating his needs.
This time belongs to me.
What a luxury.
Not really, it is a necessity to get through this illness
Though the insurance company does not see it that way.
Perhaps I shall drop my husband off for a day's stay;
By the very next day coverage will no longer be an issue
A new DSM* will be in place.

---

* *Diagnostic Statistical Manual.* Codes described here are used for billing purposes. There are specific codes that relate to Alzheimer's and reimbursement.

Lunar Moon

I sit in the office of the psychiatrist, the one who will
Do periodic medication checks. He is interested
In my background, so I tell him my story, connecting
Past and present, something I have become quite adept at.
He listens intently. I wonder if it is just part of the job
Quickly I catch myself: does it really matter?
Nonetheless, I try to be succinct, highlighting the important
Not wanting to sound whiny or martyr-like. I tell him
I am afraid of my anger and the potential damage it could do
He asks who sustains me. So overwhelmed by the question,
My mind cannot go on a search. Sustain me—it has been
Too long to even remember what that is and, as if
He could read my thoughts, he paints a picture
Of where I reside, a lunar landscape barren with craters
I am in danger of falling into if I am not observant.
There is not sufficient oxygen, nor is there an anchor.
I am adrift
I feel the sensation of not being connected, of floating
He brings me back to reality, but I am not ready
I want to linger in this place that feels familiar
Finding myself both fascinated and frightened—
Parallel to my feelings about the disease—
But our time is up.

Zen

We speak, the neurologist and I
One of our updates to keep us both informed
I tell him I often react to my husband
As if he didn't have Alzheimer's
I am well aware of what this is—my own form of denial.
I know old defenses remain in place
Defenses that worked once, now no longer appropriate
I am stuck
I have reached a plateau.
He tells me I need to go more with the flow
As the stages change, as the losses increase.
He speaks of Zen and the Buddhist approach to loss.
Going straight to transcendence is more what I had in mind
I resist the pain, the sadness
This is what keeps me blocked
This is what keeps me from going with the flow.

Guru

I am seeing an Alzheimer's guru,
At least that is how my friend billed him,
Wise, older, philosophical, and experienced with the disease.
I am skeptical; I know the drill too well.
He will tell me the usual:
Coping techniques to make my life more bearable
Advise me to feel the pain, deal with my anger.
He will monitor my answers to a list of questions
And probably ask me to rate the present quality of my life.
The inanity of the question nearly pushing me
Beyond my limits. And I will tell him
What I have told the others: "You can teach me
All the coping skills available, help me understand
My feelings, develop new strategies, but you cannot bring
My husband back." But to my surprise
He does not offer coping skills, suggest support groups,
Nor fault me for not having fully come to terms
With the situation. What he does do, front and center,
Is paint the next step in vivid colors
But not so brightly it is blinding,
Advising me to put the Safe Return bracelet on him now,
Place him on a future list for assisted living/nursing homes,
Begin to get my new life in order,
And shift my focus back to me.

Charts

She comes, Nurse Ratchett in disguise,
To aid me in my attempt to deal with the illness,
The non-medical aspects,
Upon request from the neurologist who
It seems wishes only to deal with the medical.
She does not listen to what I say
She has her own agenda.
Instead she pulls out her chart,
Admonishes me for the things I still let him do
So sure he is headed for the next stage
After all, it's there in her charts,
Scientific data for a disease that is highly individualized.
Yes, it will progress, I try to tell her, I know that,
But right now, for the moment, it is not,
So she changes tack and asks about daycare:
What are my plans?
He should be going.
Even after I tell her of the activities I've arranged
That give meaning to his day,
She will listen only to what is in her charts
And I will not turn over my husband's dignity
To her or her charts.

Another Expert

We have seen another expert on the opposite coast from us,
This time a world-class expert in the field
About a cutting-edge procedure
To find out if we are candidates,
To assess the risks, to learn the details.
The conversation turns to care
And he assures me, like our neurologist at home
That the best place for my husband is at home
That it can work, that there are classes
To support caregivers, and I silently wonder,
Do these doctors in white coats ever take care
Of anyone at home, or do they simply dispense advice
From the safety of their offices?
For it seems they know nothing firsthand about exhaustion
Or having one's home turned into a hospital environment
Or what it is like to live 24-7 with someone
Who is not present.
What is best for the patient
May not be best for the caregiver
I have seen firsthand the devastation to families,
Witnessed the exhaustion, the tears,
The inability to cope one more minute.
How many lives must be sacrificed to this disease,
Before the doctors in white coats get it?

White Coats

Today I went to see the neurologist,
Whom I am grateful to have, to talk about the future,
But he was reluctant: after all, he cannot predict the future,
Alzheimer's is not a disease of precise timetables.
I sensed his reluctance as I have before. What the disease
Lacks in preciseness the medical profession makes up for
In its precise list of discussible topics,
So, changing tack, I told him I had a therapist
For the emotional issues, what I needed from him
Was someone to tell me the truth about tomorrow
Not tell me I will make it through, or to take care of myself,
Which, he assured me, he would never do.
But not helping me in the way I need is a form of that
And I assured him he didn't have to have all the answers
I simply needed someone medically knowledgeable
To discuss the disease with, and I told him to take
A good look at me: I was not at the end of my life,
Content to make do, nor was I bailing out, but that life
With my husband had become increasingly frustrating.
I needed some kind of timeline. He listened, then politely
Reprimanded me for pushing for the impossible, for making
Myself upset, what purpose did it serve? And then I told him
What I had known all along but was too polite to articulate:
The trouble with doctors in white coats is, no matter how
Many tragedies they deal with during the day
At night they get to go home, leaving Alzheimer's behind

Imagination

Is it my imagination or is it real? I sense our neurologist
Moving away, backing off, eager to turn us over
To the nurse practitioner. After all, it is managed care
Efficient. My husband is transitioning between stages:
I am aware of new losses, mounting spatial difficulties,
Growing confusion, increased need for reassurance
I sense our neurologist does not want to talk about it.
He is briefer with me on the phone, to the point:
"If the new medication doesn't work, then he comes
Off of it." End of conversation. The tone of the office visit
Has subtly changed. Less hopeful, increasing periods
Of silence. I wonder if this is how it will be going forward.
Is this how doctors protect themselves when their healing
powers no longer serve them? Is distancing the coping
Mechanism of choice? I do not blame him
How long can one tolerate being in a situation
That is out of control? But I am still here
The other half of the patient,
And I need him to stay present for me.
I have suffered too many losses.
Medical aspects comprise only one part of this disease.
Emotional support for caregivers is a prerequisite
For the well-being of the afflicted
Physicians need to expand their area of expertise,
Enlarge their comfort zone
And treat the disease in its entirety.

Changing

Am I the one changing,
Or is it the neurologist in response to me?
Does he sense my exhaustion is more emotional
Than physical—
The wearing down of my resources,
Depleted by the monotony of my days,
By the feeling of being imprisoned
My husband in no man's land
Myself in the role I have taken on
And in the collective confinement
Of our shrinking existence?
This visit has taken a turn:
He is alternately concerned and brusque
Wavering back and forth between the needs
Of my husband and me
Clearly divided on the issue of who is the patient.

Truth

It has taken me a long while to see the light,
To understand the growing indifference of the neurologist.
In the beginning we were a team, a partnership
Going through the diagnosis step by step.
Then the focus became educational
To bring me, the caregiver, quickly up to date and on board
Followed by med checks, all part of the beginning stage.
Now firmly planted in the middle stage
The visits are few and farther between
No follow-up cards arrive in the mail
Maintenance is all we can hope for and even that is wishful.
I don't feel like part of a team anymore
More like an annoyance
Whisked in and out
In part dictated by insurance factors
Along with the truth nothing more can be done
We were dead on diagnosis.
Why did it take me so long to see?

Understanding

His neurologist cannot save him
Nor can I
An understanding I have come to
Midway into the disease
Making for a different kind of relationship.
I feel the difference in our most recent visit
I no longer question about medical advances
Ask about clinical trials
Push for a cure,
Allowing me now to hear in a new way
Making a space for his words
Both spoken and unspoken,
Objectives have shifted
Hope has been replaced by a deep sense of sadness
Helping me accept the diagnosis
Replaced by preparation for the inevitable
My husband is leaving me
Will our neurologist be next
Now that the bulk of his work is done?
I hope not
I need his strength to connect with my own.

Surprised

Surprised, that's what I am
By this most recent visit to the neurologist
The focus was not on my husband
No helpful hints, suggestions offered
Not once even mentioning the party line:
"Keep him home as long as you can."
Instead, the focus was on me
I need to start to prepare myself
For the difficult decisions coming up
Think about my life going forward
Understand my limitations,
Connect with my intuition.
For the first time I felt like a person in his eyes
Not just a caregiver.

Memo

To: Jan Mashman, M.D.

From: Your most frustrating patient who finally understood the parameters.

Message: Thanks for your patience. You know, no matter what I write in my book, I think you're great, and I'm happy to have you as our physician.

Dilemma

"He needs a colonoscopy—it is that time again."
That is what our internist recommends each and every visit,
Like a dog with a bone. I have stated my position:
I see no reason why I would put him through
The horrors of treatment if the news were bad
Much less risk the effects of anesthesia from the test.
He listens, taking it all in, seeming to understand
But on the very next visit we begin all over again.
To him I must seem non-compliant, the very worst thing
A patient can be, not to mention cold and uncaring
Issues and feelings I struggle with on a daily basis.
I wish he could come to my support group where this topic
And similar ones have been hashed around
Innumerable times. It is the safety of my support group,
Surrounded by caregivers in the same situation,
That has prepared me for my response
Given me the insight to take this stance
Years of being the good patient, years of being blessed
To have this special man as our doctor now being eroded
By conflicting opinions. Medicine is about saving lives
It has yet to differentiate or factor in the role of quality
I cannot, in good faith, risk my husband accelerating faster,
Trading off the time still available, nor do I wish
To jeopardize a relationship that, up to this point,
Has been positive. One more dilemma
One more facet of this disease to deal with.

Rehearsal

Our internist of twenty years is leaving
A retirement of sorts, a sabbatical (I hope)
Perhaps he is burned out by the demands of managed care
Perhaps it is time for a change
Perhaps he needs to do things not yet done.
It doesn't matter the reasons why
Bottom line, he is leaving. He has always been there
A unique, gifted doctor possessed of abundant sensitivity,
Caring and goodwill, a doctor who,
Upon my husband's diagnosis, became my safety net
Someone who would care for me if I became ill,
A caregiver's biggest fear. He is leaving
Just like my husband.
I feel a deep sense of sadness and longing for what was
Tinged with feelings of abandonment and anger
The same feeling I have about my husband
He is leaving and I shall compare all future doctors to him
Never letting one come close to my heart again
He tells me I will be fine
Will I?
The rational answer is yes, and I know that
The non-rational part of me thinks,
Surely this is a dream from which I will awaken
But it is not a dream, nor is my husband's condition a dream
Now I have to say good-bye to two people so dear to me
This is a rehearsal.

Peace

Somewhere, somehow, I must make peace with
My impatience with the medical community
They cannot always be the bad guys, the villains
There is a halfway point. After all, we are partners
In this disease. I am not of the generation that put blind faith
In its doctors, never questioned, never spoke up,
Nor do I have the caregiving issues of the elderly
We are in a different time and spot. Nonetheless, I know
My persistence for answers when there are none
In a world of managed care that leaves no time
For questions, much less answers, is a source of irritation.
There needs to be a new medical model for handling
This disease, an adjunct to the protocol: Understanding
And responding to the emotional sustenance needed
By caregivers to see the journey through to completion.

Experts

I want to run to the experts, whoever they may be,
wherever they may be, and ask, "What is it I should do?"
"What does life hold for me?"
But one thing I have found to be true:
The experts are not to be found in white coats,
Or therapeutic rooms,
Or over kitchen tables with friends or relatives.
The expert is inside of each of us waiting to be heard.

Tips for Communicating With Healthcare Professionals

Guides:

- *Consumer's Checkbook Guide to Hospitals*
- *Consumer's Checkbook Guide to Top Doctors*
  Published by Consumers Checkbook. Call 800/839-7283
- You will also find numerous medical web sites on your computer.

Strategies:

- Make it a priority to learn about the disease and to be well informed.
- Keep an ongoing notebook of all changes in behavior, medications, any problems, phone calls and visits to the doctor, and include the date for each entry.
- Be succinct, and come with a list of carefully prepared questions in order of importance. Leave space after each question so you can write down the response, ensuring you will not forget it.
- Borrowing from medical terminology, caregiver focus should be on verbal behavior versus nonverbal behavior when we interact with physicians. Healthcare providers, with the exception of therapists, are trained to focus mainly on diagnosis, labels, medications, directives, and outcomes. This is what is known as verbal communication. As caregivers, when we focus on empathy, acceptance, or attention (known as nonverbal communication and not to be confused with body language), we set up a barrier between the healthcare professional and ourselves.

Healthcare providers have also been taught, as part of their training, to keep a professional distance from patients in order to maintain a professional objectivity. If one is seeking empathy, acceptance, and attention, it is best to find a therapist who is trained in that area.

- Be clear in your mind about what you can expect from each specialty.
- Work out a partnership that respects both parties' needs: the need of the physician for compliance, and the need of the patient to not feel controlled or like a child.
- Remember that physicians are used to using medical terms and jargon that patients often do not understand. Ask your physician to use "layman's" terms when you don't understand what's being said.
- Do blame yourself if your relationship with your healthcare professional is less than ideal. A 2001 AMA news release showed a gap between what physicians are saying to their caregivers and what caregivers are hearing. One of the points made was that physicians need to have the knowledge and understanding to communicate effectively, and caregivers need to learn how to ask for and receive information.
- Nothing in is life is perfect, and work of some degree is always required.
- If it doesn't work out, or there is a conflict and things cannot be worked out, consider changing.
- Think of this relationship as a partnership. After all, you are the eyes and ears of the patient, and no one knows "the patient" better than you do.

Relationships

Family

The family unit is an interesting dynamic; I believe all caregivers would agree. Based on my own family and the stories I hear from other caregivers, it seems that once the shock wears off, old behavior patterns and roles return. Much of what is discussed in support groups revolves around the hurt feelings caregivers have about the behaviors of some family members. I think it is important that caregivers know when, where, and how they can and cannot expect help. This clarification, painful as it may be, means caregivers will spend less time wishing things were different and have more energy to allot to the task of caregiving. I am a proponent of family meetings where issues are laid out, expectations on both parts aired, everyone has an opportunity to say their piece, differences are worked out, and a workable plan for all is hammered out.

Our children have been a source of comfort in entirely different ways. Our son, Brian, who lives in California, has always been a wonderful listener and supporter. He doesn't hesitate to point out things I don't see and tell me his opinion, but he always offers it in a constructive way. Brian has an intuitive kindness about him. When we visit he plans special things to do and makes the visit a respite for me. His love for his father shines through in his actions and response to him. His heartbreak is also apparent, and I know he struggles with what is happening and with the inevitable loss of his father. I am his mother, and like all mothers, I want to make it easier for him or fix it. This is one time my powers as a mother fail me.

Our daughter, Laura, who lives in Alabama, is a different source of comfort. She too loves her father, and it is clear her heart is breaking also. Upon diagnosis she became driven to make sure he had a grandchild he would know and that his grandchild would have an opportunity to know her grandfather. Two of our most wonderful gifts are our darling granddaughters, Maddie Lou and Lauren Elizabeth. The love I feel for them is so intense, and the appreciation of their arrival at this time in our lives is more than I can express.

Within the family, no one's life is affected as much as the caregiver's. It's very easy to feel disappointed by one's children, and caregivers must be on guard to make sure this doesn't happen. If you are quick to label your children's behavior as uncaring, your own feelings can quickly turn into disappointment and resentment. Adult children often have a hard time witnessing the decline of a parent, and it's important to remember that each individual adapts according to his or her own timeline. It's not a good idea to put your children in the middle or in a position of having to take sides. No matter how frustrated you feel with the person you're caring for, you need to limit what you share with your children; placing them in an awkward situation doesn't motivate them to want to help you. I've seen families in which communication has broken down because of such behavior, resulting in estrangement—the last thing caregivers need or want is to lose their children.

Friends

When I think of friends an old song comes to mind: "Make new friends but keep the old, one is silver and the other gold." It is imperative that caregivers make new friends; aside from the fact that some friends will disappear, the new friends will be in the same situation and will offer another kind of friendship. I use to be annoyed about some of the friends who disappeared into the night, but with the passing of time I have come to accept it as part of the human condition. The only time I feel real annoyance is when we are about to become someone's *cause,* or someone falls all over us with words like " How can I help?" and then is never seen again.

Support Group

A support group is an absolute necessity, but the problem lies in finding the right one. Don't give up if the first one isn't the right one for you. The value of being in a group is that you learn from those who have gone before you, commiserate with those who are where you are on the journey, and welcome those who are just beginning. It's a safe haven where you can talk about all your feelings without fear of judgment or being told, "You shouldn't feel that way—after all, your spouse has Alzheimer's and can't help it." This may be true, but isn't helpful to caregivers. I'm always amazed at what is laid on the table during these meetings, with never an eyebrow raised in question or disdain. This is the best support any caregiver can receive. A support group also affords caregivers an opportunity to watch as others struggle with issues that aren't presently theirs, and is good preparation for the future. Consider going online if there's no support group in your area, if you can't find one suitable for you, or if you're unable to get out of the house.

Weekend Away

We had a weekend in Boston
Just the two of us and the kids
Having not seen their dad since Christmas
He was perfect, symptom free, on his very best behavior,
Like a child with company, and the reports that I had given
About the behaviors I live with
Suddenly rang less than true
And nicely, ever so nicely,
It was suggested that I exaggerated.
Who was I to argue?
Grateful for just a normal weekend.

Brief Moments

They've taken him out into the ocean with them
For a swim, these children of mine
Who struggle with the inevitable.
They circle around him
Protective and loving
Like he once was with them
And I lay back on the chaise
Close my eyes and feel the warmth of the sun
And for a few brief moments
He is not my responsibility
And I pretend life is like it used to be.

Sigh

"Not just occasionally but all the time."
That's what my kids tell me.
It seems I sigh
Surely they are wrong, I don't sigh
Until now with my new awareness, I catch myself.
How could I have been so unaware?
When did I slip into this despicable habit
That my whole family has brought to my attention?
I sigh it seems, long mournful sighs
When things don't go my way,
When I am tired,
When I am disappointed,
When I am at rest.
I start to apologize but my children will not hear of it
They tell me it is healthy to sigh.
When did they get so smart?

Talk Over

We talk over him as if he were not there
Our daughter the first to notice,
The first to point it out
Adding she felt badly.
We talk over him staring at the space above his head,
At least, that's how a longtime friend explained it
Admitting, sheepishly, that she found herself feeling
impatient with him.
We talk over him
At family functions, already rambunctious in nature
As if he were no longer a part
Secretly wondering if it is true,
dreading the day when it will be.
I talk over him
As if he were not there
Making all the decisions unilaterally,
Holding conversations in my head.
We talk over him
All aware of what we are doing
Saddened by our actions
Frustrated by our thwarted attempts to include him
Embarrassed by taking the low road
When, clearly, the high road is called for.

My Daughter and I

On a recent visit to my mother-in-law's in Maine,
The purpose being to introduce her to her great-grandchild,
My daughter and I shared a hotel room
While my husband stayed with his mother.
We put the baby to bed in the crib
Turned off the lights so she could sleep
And I slipped down to the bar for two sea breezes.

My daughter crawled into bed next to me,
Reminiscent of the days when she was little.
The room was dark, except for the glow of the moon
Through the window,
The conversation soft not to wake the baby,
Allowing the lapping of the waves against the shore
To be heard. The atmosphere was reassuring,
The darkness bringing with it a sense of safety,
Setting the stage for questions never asked to come forth.
She shared her concern that she and her brother were at risk
Her sadness over seeing her father's decline
The unfairness of it all, and then in what must have been
A leap of faith, she asked the question that must have been
Weighing on her mind,
Would I leave her father?

I told her the truth:
The answer was no, but at some point

I would need to seek alternate care.
She said she understood, for which I was greatly relieved.
We finished our drinks
Feeling like two schoolgirls on an adventure,
Both having taken risks and survived.
What started out as a trip to introduce the baby
Ended in an opening up of honest communication.

My Son and I

My son and I share this new relationship
The boundaries not quite worked out
Still a little awkward.
Over the phone he answers my computer questions,
Insisting they would end if I simply signed up for a course
He advises me on which credit card is the best
Tells me my phone is way too high
Listens to me when I am weary
Never judging, never offering advice, just listening.
He urges me to move to California
Where he could be of more help
But he respects my answer, "I'm not ready, yet."
And does not push. It seems like yesterday
I had all the answers to his problems—
When did the tables get turned?

Watch

I watch him, our son
As he watches over his father
Very protective, very patient,
"This way Pops, not that way."
"Let me get that for you."
It was only yesterday they were often locked
Going head to head, toe to toe
Now he tells his father that he is his role model
Bringing tears to my eyes.
How quickly a new relationship has been defined
Old hurts, resentments put aside
My son, now the one in the lead,
Has become a father to his father.

Special Child

I await the birth of our first grandchild
Coming at a much needed time in our life
There will be other grandchildren
But none like this child
So special in so many ways
Who brings hope into a world short on hope,
Who will sustain me through this ordeal.
The child whose development will parallel
My husband's losses,
We will celebrate as one learns to walk
Mourn as the other forgets,
We will be filled with joy as one says her first words
And sadness as the other utters his last words.
We will look to the future with one
And remember the past with the other
Such perfect timing, this special child and my husband
Companions on a journey with different destinations.

My Heart

My heart had been locked
Bolted down, shut and secured
Worn down by life's travails
Divorce of our son,
Passing of a parent,
Impact of downsizing,
Daughter's idiopathic kidney diagnosis,
Death of our beloved pet,
And against all odds,
My husband's diagnosis of early-onset Alzheimer's.
My heart was safe, on permanent hiatus
Protected from random assaults.
My illusions had all been shattered
A conscious decision made to hold life at arm's length
And I did just that
Until I held my grandchild in my arms
Then my heart opened
Welcoming in joy
Leaving room for hope and new beginnings.

Maddie

In the midst of darkness and devastation
Maddie came into the world
Our first grandchild
And surprised me with the intensity of feeling she aroused
In what I thought was a heart worn down
No longer capable of seeing the light
Feeling the warmth of positive emotions.
She opened my heart immediately
And slowly at the same time
Month by month delighting in her antics
Responding to her reaching out to the world
As she grew into toddlerhood,
Awakening to the infinite possibilities,
The pleasures of the world
She gave to me the gift I needed and only she could give
I saw the world through her eyes
And fell in love with life again.

Lauren

My second granddaughter, Lauren,
So different from the first,
Less intense, just happy to be here,
Content to watch big sister
Beaming a ray of sunshine with her smile so contagious
I pick her up and she responds
Smiling, cooing
How nice it is to be responded to, I'd almost forgotten
What a gift this little bundle of happiness
Her small arms around my neck reminding me of the warmth of touch
And the importance of being loved,
How lucky I am to be her grandma.

Message to Friends

Do not romanticize this illness
Or speak to me of gifts discovered
There is nothing romantic about this illness
And the gifts come at too high a price
Do not speak to me of quality of life,
For it is a quality redefined
And one that would be foreign to the person
As they once were
Do not speak to me of the Zen of Alzheimer's
Or people returned to a kinder, gentler state
The cost to the human soul is too great
To serve up platitudes is an insult
Instead, listen to what I say
The one who deals with it on a daily basis
Sit with me and understand my plight as I see it
Not as you see it
Be still with your own discomfort
So you don't need to rush in to save us both
Or present me with trivial offerings
Under the guise of caring
Just be there with me
Nothing more is needed.

Work

To my friends BA (before Alzheimer's),
You mean so much to me, more than you can ever know
Yet, you have become work
I must carry the conversation for two
Work so we appear as normal as possible
Be careful not to burden you with too much,
You have your own problems to deal with.
We have become work: a seating problem
At dinner parties, a question mark for the guest list
We really don't fit in well
Except when it is just "we" couples
But even then, we are one-half a couple
A reminder of one's mortality
Then there is the ambivalence I feel
I see your lives together stretching out before you,
The talk of travel that we all put off for retirement,
The excitement of a new stage of life,
The security of a shared history together,
And a future going forward
I am well aware I do not have that
I feel happiness for you and wish you well
But I feel sadness for us
And sorrow for what tomorrow brings.

Support Group

I sit in my support group
A safe haven where we share stories
Unload our burdens
Discuss our concerns
Support each other
There are tears, but laughter too
A sense of not being alone
At last, someone really understands.
The room is safe and warm
Reflecting the genuine concern of its inhabitants
Outside it is raining
A torrential downpour that shows no sign of letting up
A reflection of the inward part of us that we keep hidden,
Except for the times we come together.

Mirror Reflection

She is new to the support group
This woman who speaks of her husband's recent diagnosis
In optimistic terms
Sure a cure is around the corner,
Relying on the right combination of vitamins
To stave off the disease,
Planning lots of wonderful events,
Careful not to miss out on a thing,
Meticulously scheduling his day to keep his mind occupied,
Surfing the Internet to ensure his treatment
Is state of the art,
Convincing herself being young is on their side
Giving them the home-court advantage
I smile to myself as she speaks
I once was in her place
A mirror image.

Strong

"You are so strong." A sentiment I hear much too often
What does it mean?
I haven't fallen to pieces (yet)
Why is it said?
A reassurance?
And if so, for whom?
I am no stronger than any of the other caregivers
Coping with this disease
Members of my support group
Those who have gone before me
Or those who someday will be in my place
We do what it takes
Discover inner resources we never knew we had
Take it day by day
What other choice is there?

Questions with No Answers

My friend from the support group
My very first friend who threw me a lifeline,
Who knew what it was like, against whom
I measured the progress of the disease, had a stroke
It can't be true. Isn't she too young?
Isn't it just for the elderly?
Isn't that what we said about Alzheimer's?

Why?

I thought I was past the anger
Had come to terms with the disease
But now I feel the anger swell
Taking on a new freshness, a life of its own.
How can my friend at age fifty-two
Be lying in a hospital bed with a stroke?
She who has given up her life to be caretaker to her husband
Borne all the responsibilities alone
He no longer a husband or even a companion
The reason she is lying in that bed.
How were we to know? What should we have looked for?
She seemed to have reached a level of peace, acceptance
But all along a time bomb was ticking silently,
Waiting to go off.
Why must this disease claim two?

Bets

Jokingly, we place bets, wagers of sorts
These support group ladies of mine,
Most of whom have been together since the beginning.
We place bets in our minds on who will go next,
Occasionally giving voice to it, but mostly silently.
We enviously eye the new member
Whose husband is moving rapidly
While for some of us, our husbands are moving slowly,
Inch by inch
A blessing in beginning stage
Not one in middle stage
And a curse for end stage.
Like sports fans we tally up the odds
Silently placing our bets.
These are our husbands
Fathers of our children
Partners for decades
Still, we can't keep from placing our bets
Reminding ourselves black humor
Is a caregiver's survival tool
To assuage our guilt at having such dreadful thoughts.

Surprise

My support group friend's husband died
We, the ladies in the group
Received the news with mixed reactions
It was much too soon… but fortunate for both of them
To be freed from the devastation of this horrific disease
Nothing our friend would not have said or thought
In our place
After all we'd discussed it before
Wondering why those who went before us
Were not feeling set free
But the new widow, as outspoken and honest as ever,
Something we admired, warned us not to tell her
It was a blessing, or that she'd been spared
Because now she knew what the widows
Who went before knew
What the books all say
What we found so in opposition to
Our collective tiredness, our lonely psyches
That this is a terrible loss even in spite of
Years of caregiving, directing the show, taking charge
And interacting only with a shadow of what once was
And that which we achingly longed for
In our most desolate moments
What we once thought would be the ultimate relief
Turns out not to be so.

Needs

I will weather this, make it through
Like those who have gone before me did
But some days I wonder, will I?
I have so far to go, much more into the darkness of the night
I will need family even more, the joy of my grandchildren
To bring me a respite from the sorrow
The love of my children to anchor me
I will need the doctors who care for us
To be patient and understanding
When I seem demanding or anxious
I will need friends to see me through
To remind me that not all is lost
I will need my support group to lean on
So I may have a place to share my feelings
Privy until then only to me,
Weighing heavy on my heart.
I will need myself to be strong
To set an example for my children
Yet, for them to understand it is my time to regroup
And perhaps find a new identity
Or way of being in the world.
I will need to draw on the strengths
That have gotten me this far
And I will need to remember,
Even in the darkness of night,
Morning comes.

Tips on Relationships

Family

1. Weekly, or at least monthly, family meetings are essential to keep everyone on the same page. Some telephone systems allow for multiple conversations. For those separated by the miles, e-mail is a wonderful way to communicate.
2. When deciding who does what, tasks can be discussed and broken down by who does what best, then divided up and shared among family members.
3. Be prepared to deal with some unfinished business and, if needed, get outside help.
4. When a family member or friend has not seen the person for a while, it's a good idea to write a brief letter:

Dear Relative,

Since you last saw Jim/Joan, the following changes have taken place: (list). I'm taking this opportunity to let you know this so you won't be surprised. Jim/Joan still loves to talk about the family vacation we took on the Cape, and also loves to look at old pictures, so if you have any, please bring them. He/she does tire early these days, so we keep our visits short. I know he/she will love seeing you again, as will I.

5. When disappointments or hurt feelings come up, try to resolve them sooner rather than later.

    It's important to remember that each person adjusts and reacts according to where her or she is in the acceptance of the disease.

6. Keep your venting to a minimum.

Friends

When it comes to friends, an old saying comes to mind: "Friends are like pillars on the porch: some are there to hold you up, and others are there for decoration."

Support Groups

An essential tool in the caregiver's arsenal. Contact the Alzheimer's Association in your area for details: 1 800/272-3900. Don't forget about online groups for those who have difficulty getting out of the house.

Resources

- American Society on Aging (415) 974-9600
- Family Caregiver Alliance (415) 434-3388
- National Family Caregivers Association http://www.nfcacares. org or call 800/896-3650
- The Well Spouse Foundation www.wellspouse.org

Bottom Line: There is no need to take this journey alone.

Conclusion

As I conclude this book and send it to press, it occurs to me that this is yet another loss. I'm letting go of something that has been a source of comfort to me, for my eyes alone, even though my hope in sending it out into the world is that it will be of help to others. Still, a part of me remains protective. As I read through what I've written I am aware of the changes that have occurred in me throughout this journey. I will never again take life, health, family, or relationships for granted. I find myself less regretful when something ends and, instead, thankful and appreciative for the time had. I have grown ever more aware that life is cycle with beginnings and endings. And this I do know: I want to be a part of life, moving, doing, participating, and enjoying.

I still have far to travel—the hardest part of the journey lies ahead. But I feel less alone these days. To the many of you I have met during speaking engagements, to those who have been members in my support group, and to those of you who have contacted me after reading my first book, I want to thank you for your friendship and support.

It is my wish that this book will serve to lead the way, so that those who read it may not stumble or fall quite so far, and will carry with them the knowledge that they are never alone on their journey. We cannot change what has happened—only where we go.

This is a journey I never planned or wanted to embark upon, but life throws us a curve sometimes, and we have no choice but to follow along. To those of you who travel this road, I wish you the strength to make difficult decisions, an unrelenting belief in yourself, the wisdom to reach out to others, the courage to go wherever the journey may take you, and the knowledge that you are not alone.

www.unplannedjourney.com

Unguarded Moment

Sometimes in quiet moments
Caught off guard
The magnitude of it all overwhelms me.
I feel my body stiffen,
My heartbeat accelerate,
A growing sense of uneasiness
And I wonder how I will survive what is yet to come.

Trust

We are cruising,
A new experience,
Surrounded by miles of ocean
No land in sight
Each day brings the same horizon
The evenings surrounded by pitch black
Not even the moon to light the way
Leaving me without bearings
I must trust the ship to find its way to port
As I must trust myself to find my way to tomorrow.

Terrain

This is not a journey measured by miles
Or scenic signposts, or Kodak moments
Yet, we have traveled far from the safety of our former existence
To strange and unfamiliar places
Met with people foreign to us
Covered terrain that is unfamiliar and often treacherous
And never lost our way.
Though the journey is far from over
The terrain has become familiar
But we know not to be lulled into a false sense of security
For it can change without a moment's notice
How strange to be traveling this journey
Unplanned and certainly undesired
Still in many ways rewarding
The people we've met have shown us the meaning
Of the word "courageous,"
The disease has challenged out complacent values,
Realigned our priorities,
Introduced us to another world
Offered us a different path to travel
And shown us how the beauty of the human spirit
Illuminates the way.

Fine

On rare occasions when people inquire how I am,
Most often the inquiry being about my husband,
I reply, "Fine."
The expected exchange in response to a social gesture,
But I am fine
Having railed against the disease,
The injustice of it all,
Of what it has done to our lives,
Our family
All the pieces are still there
Just the puzzle no longer connects
But still I am fine
Having made the necessary adjustments,
Repositioned our lives,
And come to terms with a disease that steals
Something from everyone it touches.

Tips for Conclusion:

"I am not afraid of the *storms*
For I have learned how to sail *my ship*."
— Louisa May Alcott

About the Author

Susan Miller is a family caregiver, lecturer and workshop presenter on various facets of Alzheimer's for family and professional caregivers, and an Alzheimer's support group member. She holds an M.S. in counseling and has spent the last twelve years in the healthcare field. She is a former director of Memory Impaired Neighborhood.

Susan is available through Kaleidoscope Kare for the following:

Workshops / Lectures

Up Close & Personal: A Caregiver's Story
Looking Through The Kaleidoscope of Professional Caregiving
Understanding Family Dynamics
The Process of Change And Letting Go
The Resilience Factor In Caregiving
New Beginnings
Readings/Discussions from *Unplanned Journey* and *No Man's Land*

To contact Susan for more information about her workshops or lectures, or to place an order for a book, call (203) 762-5713.

Interested in Having Susan Speak?

Contact her at Kaleidoscope Kare
110 Pheasant Run Road Wilton, CT 06897
susangmiller530@aol.com or www.unplannedjourney.com
Or fax (203) 762-0056

Order Form

Unplanned Journey: Understanding the Itinerary

Number of Copies:_____ @ $12.95 .... _____

Sales tax 6% (Conneticut residents only)........ _____

No Man's Land: A Caregiver's Survival Guide

Number of Copies:_____@ $12.95 .... _____

Sales tax 6% (Conneticut residents only)........ _____

Both books together @ $25.00 .... _____

Sales tax 6% (Conneticut residents only)

Shipping & handling
(first book $3, additional books $1) .... _____

                                              TOTAL   _____

Name: _____

Address: _____

City: _____ State: ____ Zip: _____

Please photocopy and complete this form, then send to:

Kaleidoscope Kare
110 Pheasant Run Road
Wilton, CT 06897